By Viam

A Survivor of an Autoimmune Disease
and Chronic Illness

LEMMIE HELP YOU

VIAM

This is for them.

I wrote this book inspired by my best friend
and how much they have endured over the past few
years.

I wanted to understand my best friend,
because I knew I wasn't always told everything,
and this way their way of being utmost vulnerable
with me.

My best friend could barely hold a pen, let alone type,
so I became their scribe.

I may have written this book,
but these words,
they are all,
my best friend's
unspoken words.

Table of Contents

This book is written in three different sections. I went in writing year one thinking that was it, but then writing became an outlet for me. Year two, I was at a loss of words because so much bad had happened that I left me broken and speechless. And then year three happened, and everything changed. Things started making sense and I had so much left to say.

This is dedicated to those souls searching for what is to
come and where to go.

This is inspired by those who have been there with me
through my journey.

This book is purely written from my understanding of
what I have experienced over the last few years and to
give those snapshots of what life of a chronically ill
person is like.

My Story

If someone had told me years ago, "you will one day be diagnosed with a chronic illness or autoimmune disease", I would not have believed them. I would have said "Me?" the one that did sports all through childhood and high school, "Me?" the one that worked multiple jobs while completing a bachelor's degree full-time, "Me?" the one that thought I had it all planned out...

Imagine being thrown into a situation you never thought was possible...that was me. May 2016, I woke up and got ready for work but by the time I arrived, I felt extremely nauseated and had the biggest head pain. Who knew that this would be the start of my illness journey? I thought it would pass just like any other day that I had gotten sick but it didn't. Summer 2016 was my suffering. Constantly in and out of the Emergency Room (ER) for this head pain that would not stop. I say head pain because it did not feel like a "normal" headache or migraine, it was a constant pounding sensation that would move all over my head and never stop. Through all of this, I was visiting my General Practitioner (GP) and one visit he said to me "I think you may have *(insert name of chronic illness/autoimmune disease here)*". I went home thinking about the words my GP used – chronic illness, autoimmune disease – yes, I understood them but, me? I may have this? That was a whole other feeling of how can one so healthy have something like this? At this time, I did not believe my GP and even after my GP sent me to see a neurologist, I still did not believe that I may have something, anything remotely close to an illness.

Looking back, there were many signs leading to my diagnosis of a chronic illness/ autoimmune disease. These things are more obvious to me now in my reflections, but I just ignored it when it was happening because who wants to believe they have an illness or that they are and will be sick for life? Because it was so difficult to diagnosis, I wasn't diagnosed until it was at its worst. Looking back, December 2015 I had my first symptom, a tightness in the rib/chest area that can wrap around all the way. My GP at the time thought it may have been acidity because we could not tell what else caused that. August 2016, half my face went numb but it still was not enough to diagnose. By October 2016, my legs started getting weak and my right leg became quite heavy. Along with this I had many other symptoms that pushed my GP to refer me to a specialized neurologist. I went into the appointment believing nothing was wrong with me and left believing this neurologist had no idea what they were talking about. I moved on with my life for about two months, dealing with my symptoms and believing it was just a phase until December came along and my walking was at a point where I could not handle it. The falling, catching myself, holding the wall or such to try and move through the day.

I admitted myself to the ER, December 2016, to finally figure out what was wrong with me, why I was feeling this way and how I could make it stop. I spent 6 days at the ER, being moved to different parts of the hospital. An ER neurologist finally came to see me, completed a body scan and suggested to go ahead with an MRI with contrast to conclude. The results were 12 lesions in the brain with numerous (meaning too many to count) in the neck and spine. At this point, my mind was made up. I had to accept what was coming my way. I just didn't realize how soon that would have to happen.

With each blank page please remind yourself
to take deep breathes.

This book is heavy, with honesty and vulnerability
of the many different emotions my best friend has felt.

Remember to take a breath, a few deep breathes,
and then continue reading each page.

I was 24 years of age and this is how my story began.

These next pages in my book are dedicated to
the different parts of my life touched by this chronic
illness.

You will see these parts learn, change and grow.

Year 1

My year of learning,
what would change me,
what would leave me, &
what would grow within me.

Treatment

It was life changing.

My life changed within seconds.

Reality is, I am ill all the time.

No matter how much you read
and learn about treatments,
nothing can pinpoint exactly what you will experience,
because your experience is not the same as the person
beside you.

When people say tomorrow is the big day,
most of us think 'wedding' day or such...
And here I am thinking about
'treatment' day.

Pre-breakfast and post-dinner,
a spoon full of pills.

I am tired. I think today I have had enough. And that is okay.

Everything is at pause.
How do I even begin to understand what is happening
to me?

After all these years of feeling so strong,

I don't feel so strong anymore.

"We thought we lost you" echoing through my ears,
as I wake up from cheating death.
It is to soon, I tell myself.

When the hospital becomes your best friend,
and the receptionists and nurses know you on a first
name basis,
not because you come in so often, but,
because of the way you laugh.

Time and time again I was discouraged,
yet time and time again, I never gave up.

Sorry not sorry,
patients should <u>never</u> feel neglected by their doctor.
period.

Spoonie life is the life I am currently living
and you know what? I am okay with it.
Some days I will have more spoons than others.
It is all about balance.

I think I have reached my breaking point.

As I sit on this white bed,
I look down at my arms thinking,
where will the next mark be.

The nurse is walking towards me,
I can hear the needle whisper,
"It'll be painless"
- that's a lie I say.

Unseen scars.

Chemotherapy is a strong word.

My hair is falling,
my skin is irritated,
my taste buds are tasteless.
I don't feel like me,
even in my own skin.

I once had a doctor say to me:
"choose your suffering; if you can choose
which suffering you can deal with
only then we can help the other."

I am exhausted.
I am drained.
I do not have energy for this anymore.

I don't like the feeling of my head being caged,
'it's not a cage' says the MRI machine
- well it feels like one to me.

I went from one-month post treatment feeling horrible,
to 9 days of feeling like I had never been sick,
to down the rabbit hole again.
I am extremely exhausted.
Can we stop playing tag please illness?

Pace yourself.
Doesn't mean you start feeling better
that you forget to take care of yourself.
— I must tell my body again and again.

I giggle, I laugh, I get happy,
and at the same time,
I lose energy.
I do not have a choice
of what happens in my body.

Therapy is life changing.
Therapy kept me sane.
Therapy is a part of recovery.

This is my reality. I cannot change it.
The hospital visits,
the daily doses,
the emotional toll.
I hope in the end this was all worth it.

Remission soon please.

Relationships

*Being diagnosed with any illness
changes your relationships immensely,
whether you want it to or not.
These are things I wished all my loved ones
would understand.*

When my neurologist said to me:
"You are that oddball case, but we will get through this
together."
I realized I am in good hands.

I wanted to make you my proxy,
but we never got there.

My heart literally hurts. Can you ~~see~~ **feel** it?

I am sorry to all the people I hurt while I was hurting.

I am compromising enough, are you?

Never invalidate my feelings.
My feelings ARE MY FEELINGS.
I repeat,
MY FEELINGS ARE MY FEELINGS.

I realized some problems are like a drug.
You can have a moment of relapse to solve it
or you can find a better solution for the long run.

If this is too much, just let me know and I will let go.

I am done trying to consistently make things work with
people who don't deserve me.

I will never forget the image of an empty mattress in
my mind.
Maybe being alone is better, maybe then nobody gets
hurt.

I am not asking for anything in return,
just let me speak my words so that we can converse;
let me know so I'm not alone.

No one can tell you there is fault in you.
And if they do, they really should not be in your life.

I am so over not being loved the way I want to be.

Love me like no other,
even with my imperfections,
they make me, me.

This is how I love:
Love is such a strong and beautiful word.
It sums up emotions and feelings
that cannot be expressed in any other way
but with the singular word – love.
Love is with happiness and sadness.
Love will always be there even in tough times.
Love can make time pass so quickly.
Love is so powerful.
Love is something you feel just with a presence.
Love is something that is endless, timeless, forever.

Your love towards me,
inspires me.

I look up to you.
Everything I have learned
in these past few years
is from <u>you</u>.

I am who I am
because of how you have shaped me.
You taught me how to be a
strong independent person.

What if this brings us together even more?
I have missed you so, and I do not want to let go.

When your loved ones tell you
they are happy seeing you happy after so long.
It is one of the most gratifying feelings I have felt.

All I ask is if I give myself to you in pieces,
you see me as whole.

You get to really know someone through their
vulnerabilities.

I met an angel years ago,
she showed me what heaven is like
on earth,
when I am with her.

We lost each other within the relationship.
All the fighting left us on separate pages of our love
story.

I know who I fell in love with.
Right now, I don't feel that person anymore.
Maybe because of all the fighting
and exchanges of words that I don't feel it.
Maybe it's something else and I just don't see it yet.
Maybe because I'm just cluttered by a lot of thoughts
that keep pointing me to how I relapsed this time.
I don't know.
I have so much running through my head
that I don't know if I'm at the end of our book
or wanting to start a brand-new chapter.
I just don't know.

One thousand fights, one good day. It doesn't justify
anything

Your words became bullets...
and I became a shield.

How can I do the most good for others and do the least
harm for myself?

You meant so much to me but,
I had to let go
to save myself.

You did not help me. <u>I HELPED ME</u>.

Sometimes,
all it takes is that one voice,
to put you back at peace.

Written by my loved ones:

Your positivity is powerful; please do not let go of it.

Everything will work out in time.
We must stay strong and have faith.
Just promise to be patient with yourself
...sometimes we want to do so much
but our bodies/brain can't keep up,
so in those moments breathe
and know you are a fighter.

After all you have been through, you look really good.

You have this superpower.
You radiate happiness.
Your happiness makes me happy.
Your happiness and health is all I want.
I feel like you are reborn now.

You are a permanent ray of light in my life.

It's not fair that this is being said but you're a warrior,
if anything you always take it like a champ;
which sucks because you shouldn't have to,
but you do, it's your reality... that's... I swear,
it's like your superpower;
to take the most difficult things
and just turn them into
"it's going to be okay" kind of thing.

Pain, Suffering and Grief

I never got to mourn the loss of myself until I wrote these words.

Everyone's lives are moving,
except mine.

There is so many times I have said I am tired of living.

I don't think I can ever be comfortable in my skin again.

My eyes tell stories of silence untouched and untold.

My heart aches for you.
- they say.

White flag heart – *I am surrendering*

because

Red flag mind – *I see the warnings*

Over analyzing breaks everything good.

Everything started to feel so empty.
When will I feel full again?

I cannot remember
the last time
I felt like me.

I don't even know what pain feels like anymore.
It was killing me so much, so I changed.

Who knew that I would change for the better?

It is so easy to get lost in everything,
that I am feeling,
and forget who I am.

Some days will hit much harder than others.
I let myself feel every bit of it, because in doing so,
I am able to free myself of this pain, of this suffering.

Countless nights I feel so alone,
wondering when I will feel whole again.
Tears roll down like an endless stream,
wondering when I will shine again.
They say faith will keep you alive,
but I wonder when I will have faith again.

Tonight,
has been the most I have cried
since I was diagnosed.

"You cried as if you were grieving,"
I was told.

These feelings come in waves,
can they just sail me somewhere else instead?

I can't let time fly by. After being diagnosed I realized...
I have to cherish every moment as if it's my last
because I don't know how much time I have left.

When you want to down the bottle,
wondering if it will make you sleep for a while.

Pills in one hand, the rest of my life in the other hand.

For the longest time I thought I was going crazy,
but I must remind myself, I'm not.
My heart is too big, and I love so much,
that I give so much more. That is why I hurt.

The first time I actually felt chronically ill was
heartbreaking.

I don't know how much more heartbreak I can take.

The amount of tremors I have going on today,
and even this past week,
what is this? Why?
How is someone supposed to handle this feeling?

Pain, pain, go away, never come back again.

I lost myself.
But time seems to eventually heal all wounds,
I think.

I unstitch my heart to speak,
of the wounds I have endured.

Life lessons

Where am I going? How am I going to get there? Who is going on this journey with me?

Appreciate what's yours.
Your health.
Your heart.
Your happiness.

I have no control over what will happen.
After years of trying to control
everything I really couldn't,
I learned to just keep on smiling
because there's nothing else I can do.
Faith has given me good reason to believe
that everything will work out for the best.
Have faith when all else fails right?

I will keep going. I will keep moving forward.

I have so much to live for still.

I must have patience
in order to stay alive.

Laugh,
even on your worst days,
because there is nothing else you can do.
At least laughing takes the pain away -
takes you to sanity.

What's meant to happen is written in the stars.

Life changed
so I changed.

Loving myself again,
with all the changes that has happened,
has been hard,
though not impossible.

I will take care of myself.
By myself.

And that doesn't mean I won't ask for help.
Asking doesn't show weakness, it shows
STRENGTH,
COURAGE,
and ADMIRATION.

I **survived,** and I will keep **surviving**.

So much impacted me in my first year of diagnosis,
and living with my illness,
that is why I am so much more grateful to life now.

If I don't embrace what I am going through,
then how will I overcome it?

I am becoming comfortable in my skin again.
it's going to take a lot of time though.

I am back.
I feel like me again.
I thought my illness was changing me.
It didn't.
It was the toxicity in my life
that I finally was able to drain out.
I am back again. I am me. A much stronger me.

I forgot this whole time what being happy was.
I am happy. I found my happiness again.

I come across those who have struggled,
and let them inspire my soul.

Getting out of my comfort zone
brought me to a better place.

I am on this journey of self-empowerment and healing.

Year 2

It is not as organized as Year 1
because the unexpected happened
and my world was turned upside down.
Who thought that this would happen?

These words will try and do justice
to the emotions felt.

Disaster and Chaos

How was I supposed to foresee this?

There is no known cause or known cure for this.
To my loved ones,
please don't blame yourselves.

Everything was at a pause again.

As the seasons changed so did the news of my health...

I **definitely** did not see this coming.

Sometimes I feel like I'm living a dream,
or a nightmare really.
And I'm not sure which is worse.

Nothing could have prepared me for this.

"You may be misdiagnosed,"

said the neurologist.

I'm sick of being sick
and I don't even know what I am sick from.

I felt my heart skip a beat, or few.

Have you ever been so exhausted that you feel too
tired to talk?
This happens to me often.

I cannot wait for the day I will not have to take any
more pills.

My anger is justified. No further explanation.

If I don't ask for your advice,
don't give it.
Seriously.
Don't.

I have not been hit by a truck,
but the pain my body is feeling,
every inch of me,
feels like I have been hit by one.

I don't want to live in fear.

Fear of waking up and not being able to step,

or see,

or speak,

again.

You begin to live life as if you were dying.

But what's the emergency room really going to do for
us?
They never do anything for us.

Unspoken exchange of words.

My neurologist looked at me and said, "what do you
think we should do?"
I said, "I trust your judgment",
knowing my life is literally in their hands.

It has nothing to do with you
and everything to do with me.

What's meant to be will happen... Mostly because I
have no control over this.

Therapy Part 1

If it wasn't for therapy, I would not be writing this right now.

50% emotional health toll

+

50% numb feelings

=

100% exhaustion

I'm not ready yet.
When I am ready
you will know.

There is pain in my eyes, can you ~~read~~ **see** it?

My therapist asked me, "do you feel as though time is
passing you by?"
I respond, "Actually, no, I just feel as though I am
missing out on all the things normal twenty something
year old's do."

The sacrifices I made.

I still felt like a burden.

Just how life is for me.
Seems like whenever I finally get to a happy stable
place
shit just decides to happen.

Isn't it ironic,
I love helping people
but people seem to only hurt me?

I didn't think I could live with someone like that for the
rest of my life.
Does that make me a bad person for breaking it off?
For the safety of my health? For the safety of me?

My life will never be normal again,
but then again,
what is normal?

"You need to feel it", said my therapist.
I don't want too.
How am I supposed to heal?

“I have bigger things on my mind than you” I said.

I want someone to make me their everything.
Everything and more,
because that's what I deserve.

I have trauma from my relationships,
I'm learning to work through them,
I'm learning how much I can handle,
I'm learning the process of letting go.
"We all have some trauma;
the goal is getting through it
and moving on,"
said my therapist

I have had so many panic attacks,
because no one could help me,
understand what was happening with me.
"I must learn to breathe again", I say to myself.

Sometimes no words are better.
Sometimes all we need is silence,
with the right person.

Chemotherapy
is a medication,
treatment,
and drug;
used for many illnesses.

Honestly, I don't think anyone can ever mentally
prepare themselves for treatment.
I tried the first year and everything that shouldn't have
happened, happened.
I have no expectations anymore; I don't want to be
disappointed.

I just can't seem to wrap my head on how I am
supposed to get better
if my immunity is compromised consistently.
This doesn't make sense.

The **f e a r** of relapsing.

Heart to Heart-Breaking

I couldn't catch a break.

I don't look at myself in the mirror for days
because I cannot bare to recognize myself.

They said that with each treatment it get easier,
but why do I feel worse?

Just because you are ill, does not mean you forget what you deserve.

No one knows what it's like dating with an illness.
No one understands what it *feels* like
to be rejected
because of your illness.
No one can comprehend how painful this feeling is.
(remember, I didn't ask for this, it just happened.)

Your actions contradicted your words and vice versa.
I should have known when things weren't adding up.
You were never going to give me the full you, like I was
giving you.

It feels like a lose-lose sometimes.
I am trying to treat the illness,
yet there are so many scary side-affects,
just to get better.

How does this make any sense?
A battle against a battle?
Aren't we supposed to be on the same side?
-    *I ask my body this.*

My body feels like it's beginning
to crave the medication that has worn off.
Is this how drug addicts feel when they need more?

I wanted to be as comfortable as possible, so I took my own pillow and blanket, a book, packed healthy food and snacks but also skittles for the steroids, a water bottle, both my parents came as support too - I mean I slept most of the time but it was really nice waking up to familiar faces and honestly, I read so much about treatment *but experiencing it was life changing, for me at least.*

I take life one day at a time now. I am lucky if I can plan
for the few days ahead.

I taste metal on my tongue,
What does that taste like you ask?
Like aluminumy - like licking a battery.
(even though I never have)

When the pleasure of eating, turns to pain,
when the simplest chew
hurts
and simply becomes unappetizing.
(ordering pizza now)

The amount of things I have missed out of in life
because of the illness...

Who gave you the right to speak to me like this?
Just because I am ill?
Or is it because you think this is all a front, fake, made-up?

Tell me who would want to live like this,
with all that I feel?

"I should go"

Why?

"So I don't get reminded of who I'm not."

Sometimes there's too much truth in this world and not
enough
understanding,
kindness,
or compassion.

Nobody really understands
that you don't ever feel the same
after going through something like this.

122918

I attempted today (again) and failed.

You need to understand that I am not the same person
I once was nor will I ever be. I have changed and grown
into something much more than I ever thought I could
be.

I need a new immune system,
but sadly,
I don't think they sell those.

Any illness is bad.
I live in uncertainty everyday.
I don't know what tomorrow is like.
My treatments can cause other illnesses.
It's just one thing after another.
I haven't been able to catch a break.
To know I have a slow deterioration of nerves,
it's like a slow death.
So, I don't compare illnesses.
It's all just bad.

You: "I'm sorry to hear about your illness"
Me: "Don't be. Can't be sorry for something that is not
in your control."

I feel like I should be used to this feeling but I'm not. I
don't want to get used to this feeling.

I'm sick of going to hospitals.
Make it stop.
Please.

It's not if you're too much,
it's if I am I too much for you.
Is my health too much for you to handle?
— for this is said with any and every relationship I enter.

The truth is,
I am living a slow death.

I Am Surviving

Need I say more?

I'm still standing better than I ever did.

And other days,
I am sitting better than I ever did.

I have gained a new perspective on life
- not to settle for anything less
than what I know I deserve
and to stay positive,
to live happy, healthy life,
to cut anything toxic out,
because
this will allow me to live my truest life.

I stopped saying I used to be, and switched to
<u>now I am</u>.

If I wasn't ill, my life would be so different.

What if my illness becomes my saviour?

Faith and patience,
has got me through this,
and will continue to get me through it.

DNA doesn't make us family. Love does.

Maybe that's all I needed to do.
Take a step back
and let everything just fall into place.

"if they can't understand that now,
how can they be someone you can be with in the
future right?"

-     things my best friend told me

Always there.
Any time.
Any day.
3am or 3pm.
This is the truest form of friendship.

You are a heart in human form.
Thank you for being there for me,
when I needed you the most;
you didn't leave me.

I never feel regret anymore.
Why?
Because everything I do,
I do it for my self.
So how can I regret
if I made these choices deliberately?

Nice to hear you care,
but it's a little to late to matter now.

I appreciate everything my body
has and will
continue to go through.

I will forever choose my health over everything else.

I have no energy to fight for anything.
Not even you.
Don't take it personally,
my body decides for me.

I am my own
before I am someone else's.
I deserve nothing less of my self
and only much more
of what I can give myself.

Each time I say these words I get stronger.

Time,
we can't control it,
we can't make it move faster,
we just have to trust,
that the wait will be worth it.

I'm so tired, yet I continue to smile. I apologize to my
body, of what I keep doing to you.

Year 3

This year has been all about putting energy
only
into people who put energy into me.

Realizations and Reflections

Nothing makes sense until you look back
and give understanding
to everything that was left in question.

I forgot what it was like to lean on my best friends.
I thought I needed to do this alone.
I am thankful I realized this now.
I am far from alone.

I am stressed out
with much more
than you will ever understand.
I could care less about someone
who doesn't care about me.

"You are the one,
the one that got away."
We are all like that with someone though,
until we are with our one,
and forget that anyone else ever existed.

Many people undervalue kindness.

Why do some days just feel as if this is a slow death?
I must remind myself that it is okay to feel
the good,
the bad,
the ugly.
I must breathe.

Time tells all and shows all.
NEVER
rush this process.

I cannot go to hell and back with the same person
twice.

Your actions contradicted your words
and that's when I knew
trusting myself was what I needed to do.

It's like,
I want something serious
but to get to something serious,
I have to try with someone
to see if it even works.
But if I'm going to try
that's 50% heartbreak...
but the catch is it could lead to 100% love with
someone.

I think I'm just trying to control
what I think I can control
even though I can't control it.
Sounds ridiculous right?

Do you smile when you talk to me?
I do.

I am not going to stress about someone or something.
I don't have energy for this.

I don't think anyone understands
what it's like dating with an illness.
You can't understand
until you're in the situation
and realize
what a mess it really is.

Some days I wonder if the medications
are even working.

It's not pain, it's heaviness.
Heaviness from the inside out.
Do you know what it's like,
to feel every inch of your body
weighing you down?
This heaviness cannot be lost.
It cannot be forgotten.
It sits with me,
Heavily.

How sick is too sick?
To sick to not want to leave the bed.
To sick to not want to move.
To sick to just not want to feel,
anything anymore.

"Do you trust me?" asked my illness.
"How can I,
when I cannot see you?" I answered.

I'm always in pain
but I put up with it
because
there's nothing else I can do about it.
You just don't see it,
because
I don't complain about it.

I don't want you feeling my pain from the pain I feel.

These pills are never ending.

They say,
small improvement better than no improvement.
I say,
this feels like hell regardless,
and I've never been there.

I can't be with someone who brings their past into their
present on purpose.

All good love never seems to last.
Then again, was it even good love to begin with?

ARE YOU REALLY SORRY?
Please don't throw around "I'm sorry" like sprinkles.
You save that "I'm sorry" like a decadent dessert. You
only serve it when it's most meaningful. Everyone gets
cupcakes with sprinkles but very few afford the
decadent dessert.

-    *My hunger was speaking*

You don't know what the person,
in front of you,
behind you,
beside you,
is going through.
What gives you the right to judge them?
You don't know their story,
the hurt they have been through
the pain the have endured
the life that they have lived thus far.
Save your breath.

Woke up feeling like death.
You think you know what your worst feels like until you
feel your worst again.

Just because they seems like a good person doesn't mean that they are good for me.

I just know I'm done settling. I'm not going to settle for someone. I deserve so much more.

How ironic is it. That the person who loves so much and
gives so much
cannot find someone who will do the same for them

You can't even begin to comprehend how many times I have said "hopefully tomorrow is better" and it really wasn't.

How am I supposed to trust someone,
when my trust ALWAYS gets shattered
when I start caring about them?

Do you understand what you did?
Do you understand that this is why I have trust issues?
People throw around the word trust but the actions
never match it.

If I don't deserve it why does it always happen to me?
Or why do I end up caring about someone so much to
only get hurt?

And it's almost that time again, treatment.
My checklist:
Call nurses
Plan dates
Go for pre-tests
Emotional ride - try and prepare.

I never knew this type of sadness;
I didn't know this type ever existed.
I don't know what I'm supposed to do about my
sadness.
Depression speaks in many different ways.

I was drowning in my own tears,

And then I realized,

Only I can save me.

Remission.

The goal and the fear.

Appreciation and Acceptance

For thyself and loved ones.

You will always be home to me.

-     *To my best friend.*

I love giving guest speaking lectures about my health
journey.
If I can help one person
get through whatever they are going through,
then I know I helped make a difference.

Sometimes it's good just to be a good human,
kindness will always speak louder than you can ever
imagine.

Acceptance helps the healing process - the things my
best friend told me.

Imagine that,

each of your legs
are tied to a heavy ball and chain.
How difficult it is
to take each step on the inside
and still continue walking.

Imagine that,

you are wearing a corset around your waist
and someone is pulling the strings
tighter and tighter.
How difficult it is
to take each breath with pain
and still continue smiling.

Imagine that,

your thoughts
are consistently clouded
and you can not seem
to have any clear days in your mind.
How difficult it is
to take each thought in hopes to process it
and still continue trying.

Bad days never last.
Sometimes it's hard to think it'll pass,
but each day I have a choice to start over.

"Get home safe"
means to me that I care about you
and I want you home in one piece.
What does this mean to you?

I told you
that I have been through too much
in the last little while.
I live the life I want now.
I realized life was shorter than I really knew.

I am the roots that grow in the dark,
I am the leaves that change with seasons.

Adaptation

I live in uncertainty, and it is okay.

Sometimes the people who aren't blood related
are better than the ones who are.

You are my hero.

Things my friends tell me and I have yet to believe this.

"I wish I met you sooner" you said,
"I am happy I didn't.
I am thankful I met you now,
when I most needed too,
when it was most necessary." I said.

"To me, you are perfect too. We all have flaws.
We all have demons we need to overcome.
Love yourself more than you could love anyone.
Only then you will love someone with the purest heart
because only then you will know what love really is. "
- something someone told me

You said I have a beautiful soul and you meant it.

I felt this for the first time.

A year ago,
 I contemplated to attempt suicide.

...

A year later,
I am thankful.

I used filters for a year straight,
thinking I would be happy.
Trying to cover up what I did not want to accept.
Here I am a year later,
wishing I hadn't filtered all the pictures I took.
I wish I would have accepted myself earlier.
It was all learning though.

I didn't have a choice,
I didn't have a say
in all of this.
But look at the person in front of you now.
I appreciate me.

I've become more spiritual and looking towards God
over the past year. I think it's been helping me stay
calm in the chaos.

I have been praying for so long hoping my hair would grow back just as how it once was. I realized it will never be the same. I realized I had to accept how it is now.

This morning I felt like complete shit, like really really horrible. You could tell how badly of a toll I was taking this morning. I got in the shower cried a bit and told my self "I can do it. I have been through worse. I can get through it." I repeated this about 7 - 10 times. Continuously. I didn't stop. I just kept saying it. I got out of the shower and looked in the mirror and told myself one last time - I can do it. I got through the day. If I didn't stay positive, I would probably still feel worse than I actually did this morning. I didn't let it get to me. I fought it because I know better things are coming and I know things are going to get better. I know that hard times happen to teach me, to show me how strong I am and that I can overcome anything that does come my way to succeed. Just like you. You will achieve anything in life. Just stay positive my love. I know you can do this.

Affection.
Depends. I love the simple touch like just holding hands
or forehead kisses.
Also like when someone uses words to be affectionate
to me.

We lose our independence with our illness,
and we also become independent with our illness.
We won't know how to do it alone,
until we are alone,
because others aren't going through it.

I am a new me.
My body is still my home.
This skin is all I have.
I am finally getting closer to comfortable again.

I don't think I'll be the one to change you.
People don't change people;
people inspire or influence people which shapes the
person.
And being positive comes from within.
It's an internal change in behaviour and belief.
If you want to be more positive you will become that,
if you believe it, if that's what you desire and see
fulfilling your life.
This is how I live my life.

Can't someone else fight for me? I'm so tired of fighting
for myself,
then again,
no one knows my body like me.

The doctors never told me hair loss would be a thing.
I found out after all the chemotherapies,
immunotherapies and steroid infusions.
I found out my hair won't grow back like it used to,
and it takes twice as long.
I can't begin to explain how much hair I have lost,
and how thankful I am to have it growing back, slowly.

If I told you how much pain I carry with me,
would you still love me?

Find your RAY of hope and keep it close.

It's okay to say that I have been through a lot.

I have been through a lot.

This illness, this illness changed the way
I look at the world.

Therapy Part 2

With you it is all a learning.

I sit in therapy
With tears in my eyes.
I don't want to feel ill anymore.

I don't understand how something
that's supposed to help me
can make me feel much worse
or cause other problems.

This is so sad.

I want to let go of this feeling; I don't know how to.

They call it selfishness.
I call it healthy selfish
because I am doing it for myself
and nothing else matters more than that.

I
am not taken for granted.
LIFE
will not be taken for granted.
NOTHING
is taken for granted.

I don't regret it.
Live and learn, is what I was told.
It was all lessons that lead me to where I am in life
now.

Is time passing by you?
No.
I have learned to adjust and compromise,
to make the most of my life now.

I can't live to please anyone anymore.
It's my happiness above all.

I was finally able to forgive myself for being so hard on
myself for what I had no control over.

I blamed me for me but how could I?

My life is full of uncertainty,

So honestly, I'm not sorry if I'm asking for stability or
consistency.

- things I learned in therapy.

Therapy is a sound board.
I use it to validate my feelings.
I know who I am.
Sometimes I just need someone to validate me.

By the time you read this,
I have gone through many more infusions.

November 2019

13th set of steroid infusions; 55th dose; 3 years.

3 day infusion x 2 hours, 3000 mg total; 9-14 days later they start helping. It's a process to say the least. And they say what doesn't kill you makes you stronger, right?

...

Each time I say no more, I won't go through this again - the symptoms and side affects, yet each time I hear "if it helps, you get it done." There really isn't much choice with this, is there? If I don't get them done, the suffering gets worse, and if I get them done, maybe, I will suffer less.

Make everyday count.
Do you for you by you.
No one else.

Some people, you just have to realize, are on their own
path or journey
and maybe one day the light will guide them to the
good
but they are walking in the dark until then;
and it is not your responsibility to guide them.

Good or bad days
comes and goes
but your breath is daily.
Be thankful,
be grateful,
for something so simple,
that keeps you living.

They have the option of figuring out what's wrong and
treating themselves to get better.
Me? I am living in clouds of uncertainty. Take care of
your damn self.

All my independence is lost,
but
I am beginning to redefine independence for myself.

If I didn't get sick...
I would have moved up in my job.
I would have bought my own place.
I would have completed my master's degree.
All of it was taken away, when I got sick.

-    *How do you not see that?*

It's like when you cut up onions,
You cry but you're not sad,
that's how I feel pain.
It hurts but I'm not hurting.

My therapist replied:
"That's more than enough.
No expectations no disappointments.
Any expectations will for sure lead to
disappointments."

What a disease we have. Can't cure it. Can only treat it.
And even then, we have a 50/50 chance of it even
helping us.
We go through all these infusions, pain, side affects for
a 50/50 shot of feeling better.

Let that sink in.

It's like self-sabotage,
I want to think the worst
so when the worst happens,
I won't feel anything.

I kept telling myself I couldn't
because I don't feel good enough.
I started telling myself I can,
I just have to try,
I just have to believe.

I wonder how much of your truths were a lie.

It's like this weird twisted feeling of
this is what I deserve...
I guess.

I don't want to hurt you by showing you how much I'm
hurting.

Will I ever get used to these infusions?

Why doesn't it get any easier?

Am I supposed to get used to this?

I'm living on a prayer, hoping it'll save me.

"I'm a home body" my friend told me.
I laughed and said, "I'm a body that's always home".
-     Jokes I tell my therapist

How do you not give up? My therapist said to me.

"I'm still breathing, that means something."

It happens when it's meant to happen.
When you least expect it but most need it.

Therapist: Isn't this all so draining?

Me: You have no idea. To constantly have to think about my weak immune system, to constantly make sure I don't get sick – I feel like I'm crazy using my hand sanitizer 24/7. I don't feel like the normal ____ year old.

Therapist: I can't imagine, but I hear you trying your best to take care of yourself.

Me: If I'm not going to take care of myself, who else will?

If I speak about you during my therapy session,
you're either pretty special
or pretty toxic.
Choose wisely which one you'd like to be
because that's in your control.

My illness does not define me.

I define my illness.

I define me.

When I say it to you,
when I say it out loud in this room,
I know it becomes real,
and that I have to finally face it.

Lost... And Found

Myself.

All these presentations I give of myself,
they aren't just for you,
they are for me.
With every word I speak about myself,
I understand me more.
My body,
my heart,
my soul,
my feelings.
Mentally, physically, emotionally.
It is all creating me into who I am now.

-    *The new me.*

It's hard reading all of this sometimes
and looking back at what I am going through.
Because I don't realize
HOW MUCH
I have really gone through.

-    *How much is too much?*

When do I ever complain about what I am going
through?
I don't. I tell myself I will get through it and I do,
even with the pain, the tears, constant battle in my
head.

-    *I get through it.*

My patience was consistently tested this year. And I
know it'll continue to be.

-    *Don't ask me how I am so patient,*
     when you should be able to feel why.

I do hope you find love again,
with someone so caring,
that gives you everything you need.

-    *I will always care for you.*

I am going through a lot of things
that are still very hard to process
and I am trying my god damn best
with every inch of me that I can.

-    *The struggle is real, very real.*

The truth fucking hurts
and it is better than a baseless lie.

-    *Honesty is the best policy.*

Struggled badly last year with that.
Tried so hard to control something
I didn't understand and couldn't.
This year I learned to let go
and let things fall into place by themselves.

-    *You cannot control what's not in your
hands.*

I think everyone I have met,
and will continue to meet,
happen at a certain time and specific place
for a reason.

\-   *Everything seems to make sense in due
time.*

You,
must accept me
for me and all of me.

-    *For I have accepted myself, for me.*

If I didn't get to where I wanted to be,
maybe I wasn't meant to get there at all.
Maybe I was meant for other things?

-    *Things will fall into place.*

How am I supposed to continue living, if living means
living with all these symptoms?

-     *I must come to terms with this.*

Nothing ever came easy to me. Why would I think it
would start to now?

-      *Haven't I been through enough?*

Most mornings I wake up nauseous,
in pain,
not wanting to leave my bed.
Yet I still do. I continue living.

\-   *My resilience is my strength.*

It takes hard work and dedication
to have a positive outlook on life
but
this positive outlook is what keeps me going.

- *Things I tell myself to continue living.*

It hasn't been easy;
I wake up everyday and constantly, continuously tell
myself that
I am going to have a good day.

- *this should come naturally but it doesn't.*

I have to be the best me for me
no matter how badly I am struggling every day
because it's the only way I'll get through this.
-     *What more can I do?*

"I appreciate you so much."

*- things my friends tell me; and I still wonder why,
because I am just being me.*

I just never give up,
on myself or others.

-    *Giving reasons to continue, always.*

We encountered. We lost. We reconnected. We found.

-    *Us*

Everyone else was a lesson. You're the blessing.

-   Some relationships are everlasting.

"You make me want to be a better person."

-    *Things my friends tell me.*

I've done enough good
that if I die tomorrow
I know I'll have enough happiness
to last me a death time.

-    *Get it?*

You
treat yourself,
spoil yourself,
love yourself,
to forget the horrible feelings of
pain, anger, sadness.

-    *It's healthy enough for me.*

You have a Heaven-sent angel face.

-	*I can't help but smile when I look at you.*

One muscle.
One hundred emotions.

-     *The heart.*

I am trying to forgive pieces of me hurt by others.

        -    *Letting go is all I can do.*

No one is ever going to understand me like I do.
No one is ever going to take better care of me than me.

-	*Fact.*

"You just have a way of making people realize who
they are,
who their true self is."

-     I've been told this, many times.

The stars bleed yellow to paint the night sky,
I bleed red to paint what is unsaid.

-    *All the bottles of blood I get taken out.*

Everything seems to happen for a reason,
everything falls into place when you least expect it;
just wait,
be patient
and have faith.

-    *Something I learned to accept over time.*

"I never give up; I never stop believing in myself"

- *a lesson a friend said they learned from me.*

It's all happening and going to happen so fast.

- *Next treatment now? Where did the year go?*

You're never going to grow if you hold on to what's in
your past.

-    *Closure is necessary most times, not all.*

If it doesn't scare you it's not right.

-    *Things I've learned from this illness*

And I know.
It's just all anxiety for 100 reasons,
just not one.
And that's just how it is for someone who is ill
and knows
not to have expectations
because nothing ever goes right.

\-   *Better to save my heart than feel pain.*

"Be at peace" my illness said
"How can I?" I replied.

-     *The inner self-dialogue*

I do it and then I deal with the aftermath of it. Because I'm not going to stop living my life.

-   *I am to young to give up on myself.*

I've been looking for you, did you miss me?

-    *The bottles of pills.*

My whole life I have done things for everyone else.
I'm done with that.
I'm doing everything for me now.

-    *the promise I made to myself.*

"I am in awe of how you carry yourself through all
this."

-      *things my friends tell me.*

There's something special about a voice, right?
Like it's a different type of intimacy
listening to someone,
like a sense of calmness.

-    *I can't see you but I feel you.*

This is the year of closure.

-    *All the answers I have been waiting for.*

Why don't they teach health and illness
in elementary or high school?
Why isn't it apart of the norm to speak of illnesses?

-    *Things I have questioned now more than
ever.*

How can I help?

-    *the question I want to hear but no one asks.*

I never realized how beautiful this place could be.

-      *the hospital.*

I am so much more than my illness.
Even on my worst days.
Even when it feels like it's eating me alive.

\-   *I am so much more than this illness.*

This illness,
this illness changed the way I look at the world.

\-   *My perspective.*

~~Remission soon please.~~

Healing soon please.

Acknowledgements

Thank you to my:

My Therapist,

My Neurologist,

My Nurses,

My Pharmacists,

And of course,

My Loved Ones.

Calvin "Kalvonix" Tiu, I cannot thank you enough; not only for being the editor of my work, but also you have inspired me in the art of being me, sharing my story, and realizing there is so much to give the world – even if it is to one person. Your dedication with inspiring others and reducing stigma in mental health through your music has connected many across the world. Continue being you. Calvin has a bachelor's degree in English and a minor in counselling.

For contact: calvintiu99@gmail.com

You can check out Kalvonix's music on Spotify, Apple Music, YouTube and other major platforms.

Laughter Peacefully Breathtaking

Simply, thank you.

RAY

If someone asked me what growth was,
it is both of you.
What has blossomed from your storms
has inspired me to continue,
always.

Special Kindness

You taught me the law of attraction
which has led me to writing this book.

My Truest Resilience

For every time you dig yourself out,
your courage and strength inspires me.

Just Admirable

For everything we have been through together,
you constantly show me what it means to persevere
time and time again.

This book encompasses excerpts from the life of one with a chronic illness, autoimmune disease and an invisible disability. This is for those struggling to help themselves, or to help others understand what this life is like to live. In no way does this do justice to everything one goes through, but this is to give a glimpse of what it is like and what can be endured.

As you read each line, I hope you can feel what is meant to be felt – whatever that feeling may be, and I hope you realize you are not alone in this.

The most powerful thing I can do is share a part of my past with you. If you can accept me after hearing everything I have been through, how it has affected me and how it has shaped me into who I am today, only then will you understand me.
Only then you will see me as whole.